How Can We Save Our Marriage?

A SELF-HELP GUIDE FOR TROUBLED MARRIAGES

TONY AND BETTY DADY
Founders of the Catholic Marriage Centre
North Wales

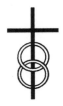

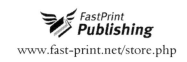

www.fast-print.net/store.php

HOW CAN WE SAVE OUR MARRIAGE?
Copyright © Tony & Betty Dady 2013

A catalogue record for this book is available from the British Library

ISBN 978-178035-671-6

Excerpts from Papal and Vatican documents copyright © by the Incorporated
Catholic Truth Society and used with their kind permission.

Excerpts from *Catechism of the Catholic Church* (CCC) (London: Geoffrey
Chapman, 1994) are reproduced by kind permission of Continuum International
Publishing Group, London.

All Scriptural excerpts are from *THE JERUSALEM BIBLE*, copyright © 1966 by
Darton, Longman & Todd Ltd and Doubleday, a division of Random House, Inc.
Reprinted by Permission.

First published 2013 by
FASTPRINT PUBLISHING
Peterborough, England.

Dedicated to the Sacred Heart of Jesus

*Through the Sorrowful and
Immaculate Heart of Mary*

And

The many married couples we have ministered to

Contents

Introduction

'God created man in the image of himself,
in the image of God...' (Genesis 1:27a)

Presumably you have picked up this booklet because you are finding that you are experiencing problems in your marriage. Do not be surprised! After all, we are all wounded and sinful creatures trying to love our God and those around us, and we do not find it too easy, much of the time! As Fr Thomas Merton wrote *"As long as we are on earth the love that unites us will bring us suffering by our very contact with one another. Because of this, love is the resetting of a body of broken bones. Even saints cannot live with saints on this earth without some anguish, without some pain at the differences that come between them."*

The Catechism of the Catholic Church (CCC) points out that marriage is under the regime of sin, and we all experience evil around us and within us. *"This experience makes itself felt in the relationships between man and woman. Their union has always been threatened by discord, a spirit of domination, infidelity, jealousy and conflicts that can escalate into hatred and separation."* (CCC n.1606).

"...the disorder we notice so painfully does not stem from the nature of man and woman, nor from the nature of their relations, but from sin." (CCC n.1607). To heal the wounds of sin, the graces received from the sacraments of Confession and the Eucharist are essential.

Sadly, when you experience problems in your married relationship they feel so much worse because the relationship began with close, intimate, warm, loving feelings which you rightly expected to continue for a lifetime, and which now seem to be vanishing. Maybe you have lost hope that these feelings can ever be recaptured, and your relationship restored. Nevertheless, don't lose hope; when both you and your spouse wish the marriage to be saved and healed, it can be, with God's help and your prayer and effort! Even if your spouse seems unwilling to do anything, the graces of the sacrament, prayer and your efforts will still improve the relationship.

Marriages can of course be under severe stress through circumstances over which you both have no control, like unemployment, poverty, accidents and bereavements. This calls for great love, understanding, compassion and maybe recourse to outside professional help. Within the marriage, problems caused by medical conditions, finance, children, addiction to alcohol, drugs or pornography, and domestic violence, are often very difficult to deal with, and will almost certainly need the appropriate professional help.

This booklet, however, deals with areas where we feel you can do much to heal, save, rebuild and enrich your own marriage. We have found that it has been a great help to those experiencing marriage problems if we explained what we felt was happening in their relationship, in order that they can see what needs to be done. Our explanations, instructions and suggestions are the result of over twenty years of 'hands-on' marriage counselling and teaching, so we have adopted and distilled these techniques to help you in this booklet. We start, then, with the premise that the key to improving, restoring or healing your marriage is to try to see what is actually happening in the relationship, and identify what may be causing this. It follows, therefore, that this is where your efforts and your spouse's efforts need to start! Because understanding what has led to the problems in your marriage needs to be clearly understood before you can begin to bring healing, we have given detailed descriptions of the more important and common areas of relationship breakdown and the causes. Continuing from the description, we point to steps that you may take to deal with and heal the situation. **We have printed these 'helps' in bold type for easy reference.**

As marriage between baptised Christians is a sacrament, in which the material sign of the sacrament is the mutual exchange of true love between wife and husband, Christ's love is *made present* in the sacrament. Therefore, you and your spouse are given the grace to love each other with the love that Christ has for his Church. *"This grace proper to the sacrament of Matrimony is intended to perfect the couple's love and to strengthen their indissoluble unity."* (CCC n1641.**)** Whatever the problems are, pray for the graces of your sacrament; and remember that prayer must undergird all your efforts to restore or improve your relationship. We will look more closely at the importance of this, and the importance of forgiveness in your marriage, in Chapter 1 - 'The Spirituality of Marriage'.

In what may sound somewhat of an over-generalization, it has been said *"that all relationship problems in adult life stem from problems in our childhood."* We believe that what this is saying is that the wounds received as a child from parents and other authority figures, condition reactions in the here and now. It appears that we all need *inner healing* to a greater or lesser extent; that is, healing of the 'wounded child' within us. Therefore, your life with your parents, or whoever raised you, is the root and trunk of your life. Whatever behaviour manifests itself in the present derives from those roots; so, although the causes for present marriage problems have clearly to be given full consideration, the *root causes* need to be searched for mainly in your *childhood*. Inevitably, hurts and wounds received at a very early age, although recorded in our unconscious, may very well be forgotten now in the present. Therefore, some detective work may be necessary to trace these back from your exhibited patterns of behaviour in your relationships today. There is a spiritual element involved here too because, when you were wounded in the past, you almost inevitably judged those persons (usually your parents) consciously or unconsciously, and this has implications. We will deal with this in Chapter 2 - 'Our Wounded Past'.

In addition to these wounds you received in your childhood, your brain permanently recorded and stored all the memories of your experienced childhood emotions, feelings and reactions that resulted from what your parents said or did. These archaic emotions and feelings are frequently triggered by what your spouse says or does, and you need to look at whether, in your relationship, you respond in an 'intentional' and 'thought-out' way, or 'automatically' in a 'knee-jerk' reaction. We examine this more fully in Chapter 3 - 'Confused Emotions' and see how these reactions can be recognized, and controlled if necessary.

Little progress will be made in restoring your marriage unless you can communicate clearly and calmly with your spouse! Communication is two-way - you *both* need to hear and understand what the other has said, and be able to respond clearly and unemotionally. Pope Benedict XVI has recently said: *"Cultivate this valuable habit of sitting together to talk and to listen to each other, to understand one another again and again in face of the surprises and difficulties of the long journey."*

We will suggest techniques that will help you to do this safely; and we will emphasise the importance of sharing your feelings and emotions with each other, in Chapter 4 - 'Communication'.

Who or what do we put first in our marriage? If our priorities are disordered from the start, or become disordered during the marriage, almost certainly the relationship will suffer and, if not reordered, will probably be damaged beyond repair. We look at potential problems and how to be aware of them in Chapter 5 - 'Priorities in Family Life'.

In our last chapter, Chapter 6 - 'Gender Differences', we look at how sexual differences, due to different brain functions as well as physical differences, can affect you in a number of ways. These, as in many other areas mentioned above, can cause serious difficulties in your relationship if ignored or not understood.

The Church's teaching on marriage may seem almost impossible to live. Jesus, however, said: *"With men this is impossible, but with God all things are possible."* If we surrender our lives to the grace of redemption, it is truly awesome to know the joy, freedom, wonder and excitement that comes from living and loving according to our true dignity as men and women made in the image and likeness of God. It is truly possible for husbands and wives to experience the restoration of proper balance and mutual self-giving in their relationships. This is the Good News of the Gospel. The Holy Spirit is in our hearts; that Spirit of love, which makes the cross of Christ fruitful in our lives and enables us to live the full truth about the sacrament of marriage.

Finally, there is an appendix on 'Fertility Awareness', giving details of various ethical methods of Family Planning, in accord with the Church's understanding and teaching in this area.

Tony and Betty Dady
Feast of St.Benedict 11th July 2013

1. The Spirituality of Marriage

'For this reason a man must leave his
father and mother' (Ephesians.5:31)

LIVING THE SACRAMENT

St. Paul, in his letter to the Ephesians, was the first to lay the real foundation for the understanding of marriage as a sign or sacrament of Christ's love, when he said:

"For this reason, a man must leave his father and mother and be joined to his wife, and the two will become one body. This mystery has many implications; but I am saying it applies to Christ and the Church." (Ephesians 5:31-32)

Marriage is one of the seven sacraments of the Church and, as such, it is important that couples know how the Catholic Church sees the sacramentality of marriage, and how they are called to live that out. Therefore, in this chapter, we will describe how marriage fits into the broader understanding of our faith, and how the spouses are called by God to live spiritually, emotionally and physically as Christians in their marriage. We will look at the spirituality of marriage as the Catholic Church sees it, enriched by the insights of Blessed John Paul II's 'theology of the body'. Marriage is an exclusive, indissoluble, intimate union of life and love entered by man and woman at the design of the Creator for the purpose of their own good, and the procreation and education of children. Christ has raised this covenant between baptised persons to the dignity of a sacrament. We strongly recommend that all couples read the excellent overview of the sacrament of marriage in the *Catechism of the Catholic Church* (CCC nn.1601–1666, & nn.2331–2400) and, in addition, *Familiaris Consortio*, regarding the role of the Christian family in the modern world, by Blessed Pope John Paul II.

It is said that we can't really understand Christianity if we don't understand and keep in mind the 'great mystery' involved in the creation of mankind as male and female and the vocation of both to marital love; that is, the real truth, purpose and meaning of our sexuality. (Cf. *Letter to Families*, n.19). In the Trinity, God is a *life-giving communion of persons.* ('Communion' means 'in union with'); so, the three *persons* of the Holy Trinity are in a *perfect union of love*, one with the other, and are *life-giving.* God wanted to make the mystery of the Holy Trinity in some way *understandable and visible to us,* so we are told he created us in his own image and likeness. God's plan is that we image him in our own loving communion with our spouse, which extends beyond just our bodily union, to a union of our very beings – *body and soul.* It is in this aspect we make visible God's invisible mystery of life in the Trinity. This mystery is that God is LOVE. If we are created to be a sign of the Holy Trinity, we are called then *to love as God loves in the Trinity,* which is as a *life-giving communion of persons in love.* However, as human beings created as male or female, we are called to do this through our sexuality.

Marriage, we have said, is a sacrament. Now we can speak of a sacrament as a *material sign or action that draws our attention to some profound, spiritual truth.* It does this because in some way it resembles that spiritual truth. Moreover, in a sacrament, the acting-out of the sign makes the spiritual truth present. Therefore, in the sacrament of marriage, in the context of our Christian faith, *the couple's love of each other is a sign that resembles, and an action that draws our attention to, three profound, spiritual truths.* That is, the love and communion within the Trinity, the love of God for his Chosen People, and the love of Christ for his bride, the Church. Through the material sign of the sacrament, that is, the mutual exchange of true love between husband and wife, Christ's love is *made present* in the sacrament. The couple are given the grace to love each other with the love with which Christ loves his Church; that is, their love becomes transformed, perfected and grace-filled.

Clearly, if you are not living the 'sign' of the sacrament, as we describe it below, the marriage will be beset with problems small and large, as God's will for you is not being recognised and followed. Therefore, if you are experiencing difficulties, problems or even threatened break-up in your marriage, you will need first to see where you are failing as an individual or as spouses to recognise and live a truly Christian life. Are you regularly receiving the Sacrament of the Eucharist? If you are both Catholics, you will almost certainly have been married during the Nuptial Mass, where in the Eucharist the memorial of the New Covenant is realised. *"The New Covenant in which Christ has united himself forever to the Church, his beloved bride for whom he gave himself up."* (CCC n.1621). It was, therefore, fitting that you should have sealed your consent to give yourselves to each other through the offering of your own lives by uniting them to the offering of Christ for his Church made present in the Eucharistic sacrifice. By receiving the Eucharist, by communicating in the same Body

and the same Blood of Christ, you formed but 'one body' in Christ. (Cf. CCC n.1621). How vital then, it is for your marriage to renew this grace by regularly receiving the Eucharist.

As we look at the more important potential areas of trouble in marriages we will suggest various ways to deal with these, ways to solve problems and ways that various techniques should be able to help you. However, underlying all of these helps, there needs to be the realisation that each calls for you to act in love and to be truly Christian! Are you regularly receiving the Sacrament of Confession? When you are not being truly Christian, you should consider whether this requires receiving the full benefits of sacramental Reconciliation. All of the techniques will certainly be more fruitful if carried out with God's graces and prayer.

Marriage, however, has been affected by the fall. In our fallen state, we need help in breaking out of our 'egoism', our selfishness, our 'self-absorption', the pursuit of our own pleasure, etc. In other words, we need to *learn how truly to love!* This is the only path to salvation; and what better path than through marriage, a vocation that demands total, self-giving love?

What, then, is total, self-giving love? As we are created in God's image and likeness, we are called to act as God acts, and to love as God loves. Jesus exemplified God's love by his sacrifice on the cross. He clearly *freely chose* to die on the cross, and this was an *informed decision*, as he wished to do his Father's will. The sacrifice of his life for us was a *total self-gift,* without reservation, and it was *faithful* and *permanent,* for the effects of his sacrifice extend into eternity. Finally, the death on the cross was *fruitful and life-giving,* as this act was for our salvation. These are the four most important characteristics of God's love: it is *free, total, faithful and fruitful.* Therefore, if we are to love as God loves, then our love should reflect these four characteristics.

When we come to marry, we have *freely* made that decision based on the knowledge and love that we have of each other. In exchanging our marriage vows, we promise to *freely* undertake the obligations of marriage. These are to accept the 'goods' or blessings of marriage: *faithfulness, indissolubility* and *fruitfulness* (being open to procreation). We are also asked if we are ready, freely and without reservation (that is, *totally*), to give ourselves to each other in marriage. In short, we promise to love each other as God loves us, in total, self-giving love. When this love is consummated later in the genital, 'one flesh' sexual union of the marital act, an unbreakable bond between the spouses is established; and for the baptised, this bond is sealed by the Holy Spirit and becomes indissoluble.

For many, the most difficult area to achieve this total, self-giving love to one another, and a consequent potential cause of much friction in marriage, especially between a Catholic spouse and one of a different denomination, is whether or not to use contraceptives. *Contraception* is holding back or preventing total self-gift to one another, altering the sexual act and making it something other than total self-surrender. This means that, in the terms of our definition above of God's love, it is not truly loving. In turn this implies that, in this area at least, we would in fact be *using* each other as a means to an end to enjoy sexual pleasure. In refusing to give ourselves to one another as potential mothers and fathers, we are engaging in what is only an *apparent* act of self-surrender. Since the sexual union is no longer the expression of *total* gift, it is no longer an expression of the *true love* to which we are called, that is, loving as Jesus loves. Although we may not realise it, the act has become, in effect, both a *contradiction and a lie.*

This is why the encyclical on Human Life condemned *"any action which either before, at the moment of, or after sexual intercourse is specifically intended to prevent procreation, whether as an end or as a means."* All methods of contraception, including oral contraceptives are, therefore, morally unacceptable and, if culpable, we could be sinning. *"So the Church, which is 'on the side of life', teaches that 'each and every marriage act must remain open to the transmission of life'."* (CCC n. 2366).

As responsible parents you may, for just reasons, wish to regulate the timing and number of your children. It is, however, your duty to make certain that your desire is not motivated by selfishness but is in conformity with the generosity appropriate to responsible parenthood. Cf. (CCC n.2368). Regulation of births by periodic continence *"based on self-observation and the use of infertile periods, is in conformity with the objective criteria of morality."* (CCC n.2370). That is, you can still truly love one another, and still reflect *all the four characteristics of God's love.* Although you may be restricting intercourse to the wife's infertile period, there is *no actual impairment of the sexual act;* you are doing nothing to prevent it being fruitful and, although it is extremely unlikely, the act always remains *potentially fruitful, or life-giving.* Ethical methods of birth regulation are discussed in the Appendix at the back of the book. *"These methods respect the bodies of the spouses, encourage tenderness between them

**and favour the education of an authentic freedom."
(CCC n.2370).**

**Natural family planning or fertility
awareness, however, takes prayer, trust in God
and one's spouse, self-control, honest and open
communication, and willingness to sacrifice for
each other. Nevertheless, these things do not
harm love; these things *are* love.**

The Church describes marriage as a *vocation.* *"God
inscribed in the humanity of man and woman the vocation,
and thus the capacity and responsibility, of love and
communion."* (CCC n.2331). We are all *called to holiness,*
and it is saying that marriage is one specific path to this
holiness. The daily actions that comprise married life
are the actions that can lead us to holiness, through
carrying them out in love and in accord with God's
plan for marriage.

In our Catholic tradition, the spouses themselves
are the ministers of the sacrament, the priest being the
Church's official witness. Thereafter, our entire
marriage should become a sacrament we minister to
each other, daily. In practical terms, continuing from
the wedding, *whatever goes into the building of a happy
marriage and a happy family is authentic ministry* between
us. We can minister to each other spiritually,

emotionally and physically. For example, most importantly, we will pray together, we will encourage and strengthen each other's faith, reveal ourselves to one another as we really are, counsel and advise one another, affirm one another and build each other up. We can comfort and heal one another, ease one another's burdens, mutually exchange the gift of ourselves to one another and exercise the mutual rights to one another's bodies.

Ministry is 'service', the basis of true unconditional love, which should be at the heart of every marriage. We will look at two important spiritual aspects in this chapter: prayer and forgiveness.

PRAYER

You surely will wish to pray for your spouse, your marriage and any specific problem areas as and when they surface; in addition, however, it is an important element of your ministry to one another to engage in prayer together as a couple before God. This is important, because Christ is truly present at the centre of your covenant of love. *"For where two or three have met together in my name, I am there among them."* (Matthew 18: 20). You are the *two!*

You are both called to lead each other to holiness, so you will both wish to place all your requests for your marriage and family needs before God. Before doing this, you will see the necessity to resolve all conflict before the time set for prayer, and to seek and give forgiveness for any hurts between you. It is a powerful and beautiful prayer for continued intimacy, daily to renew and keep the vows you made before God; it could just be simply saying: *"I renew my vows to you, till death parts us."* It is a duty for you as parents to pray also for your children, and this is especially so when they are in wrong relationships.

If you are not actually praying together in your marriage now, it would be worthwhile to examine why this is so. Often it may be because you don't feel intimate enough, and probably uncomfortable or embarrassed because you haven't experienced praying like this before. However, if you have never even given serious thought to the idea, or you say you have no time to pray, or whatever the reason may be, *now* is the time to start, and you will surely find it rewarding. It is best to make a *commitment* to God and one another to pray together regularly, that is, to make a *decision.* You certainly can't rely on *'feeling'* like praying.

To help you to get started, we suggest that you should agree suitable and *specific times* for your prayer together. *At the beginning of the day:* for the graces and blessings of your sacrament, and to renew your marriage vows to each other. *At the end of the day:* to examine together the day that is closing, and thank God for all the blessings received; also to seek and give *forgiveness* to each other for any hurts received. Ideally, it would help to make it a habit to have a focal point or place to meet and pray and, perhaps, light a candle to help you to focus your prayer.

There is certainly a biblical principle that the *husband has the responsibility* for the spiritual development and religious training of the family, leading them to an increase in holiness. So it is a good idea for him to initiate prayer at the agreed times.

When there are children in the family you will also need to have a separate time for family prayer; the form and time will naturally depend on their ages; however, it is not only important for the children, but it will strengthen your own

prayer life together. *"Based on the sacrament of marriage, the family is the 'domestic church' where God's children learn to pray 'as the Church', and to persevere in prayer."* **(CCC n.2685).**

FORGIVENESS

Whenever we are sinned against or hurt, we make a decision either to forgive or not to forgive, and thereby harbour resentment and build up bitterness within us. *Forgiveness is mandatory.* It is a non-optional principle of life taught to us by Jesus. The Father will forgive us only if we forgive those who offend us. This is not that God is punishing us, or withholding forgiveness from us, because we have not ourselves forgiven others; but rather that we have, in effect, rendered ourselves incapable of receiving forgiveness. The Divine mercy is powerless before those who refuse to acknowledge that they have sinned, and who refuse to forgive others. We must always take the initiative and we must always be in the right relationship before we worship. Jesus is our model for forgiving others, and we must forgive as often as necessary. The parable of the unforgiving debtor highlights what God has forgiven us, and what we are asked to forgive, in turn. (Matthew 18:23-35).

Forgiveness is giving up all claims on the one who has hurt us, and letting go of the emotional consequences of that hurt. All resentment must go. We must take the first step of healing the relationship, and we mustn't wait for repentance from the other. We have to give up all rights of revenge, because we are called to give mercy, not demand justice, and this runs counter to all that our society teaches! Vengeance and retribution are not our responsibility; God (and possibly the Law), will deal with any consequences. Forgiveness is never conditional and can't be earned; it is not pretending something did not happen, nor is it indifference to something that did; neither is it just putting up with something or condoning something wrong. We must be clear here to condemn the sin, but love and forgive the sinner. There may, however, be discipline and/or restitution required! *If we are seeking forgiveness we must express sorrow, accept responsibility and ask forgiveness for the specific offence.*

Why don't we forgive? Probably because we may harbour bitterness or hold grudges, or we may have a history of hurt in our life. Fear of making ourselves vulnerable and being hurt again is also a possible reason. Jealousy may prevent us, because we don't feel forgiveness is deserved, or maybe we feel we can't continue forgiving a person who continually offends us, and we say 'they'll never change'; *but we must not judge, just forgive!*

The consequences of un-forgiveness are considerable and dire, because spiritually we are violating God's law and will suffer the consequences of turning from Him. This requires us to seek the sacrament of Penance or Confession with contrite heart, to restore us to God's grace. Psychologically we are in bondage to those we have not forgiven, because they affect and control our lives. We can suffer the same hurt time and time again, whenever we see or think of the person who hurt us! We can suffer physically, too, because un-forgiveness and bitterness may cause many of the illnesses associated with stress.

It is important to recognize the difference between *forgiveness* and *reconciliation*. As Christians, we work towards forgiving everyone; some people, however, are unrepentant. We can only be reconciled to people if they acknowledge the harm done to us and have fully faced the consequences of their actions or sin. Restoration of relationship, even with the most horrendous hurts, is possible, but only if the person has shown a deep, accountable and repentant change.

Having looked at the importance of forgiveness in your life as a Christian, there is

little need for us to stress how forgiveness or un-forgiveness will greatly impact on your marriage relationship. In marriage, if you are unforgiving you may suffer in all the ways mentioned above, and married life will be intolerable. You will be unable to develop a deep, lasting and intimate relationship as you destroy the potential for intimacy, especially in communication, where your spouse will be in constant fear of offending and always feeling vulnerable. The rule in marriage is to forgive as soon as possible after a hurt; and never let a hurt go unresolved or unforgiven overnight. *"Do not let resentment lead you into sin; the sunset must not find you still angry. Do not give the devil his opportunity."* (Ephesians 4:26-27). You will find that forgiveness, practised regularly in marriage, leads to increased intimacy and love, as it generates greater communication and vulnerability. To love despite faults and failings engenders greater love in return. Remember, love keeps no record of wrongs!

Clearly, if you find you are having difficulty in forgiving your spouse, you need to act now! Not only do you need to take the steps we outline here but also, importantly, you probably need to seek sacramental Confession as you are contravening God's law by holding un-forgiveness. In receiving this sacrament of Penance with a contrite heart and religious disposition, feelings of peace and serenity of conscience inevitably follow. Cf. (CCC n.1468). However, this outpouring of mercy cannot penetrate your heart as long as you have not forgiven those who have trespassed against you. Cf. (CCC n.2840). A sincere confession can help you feel more accepting of your spouse, and make you more likely to be able to take the difficult decision to forgive more readily another time.

It is very important to recognize that forgiveness is initially a decision and not a feeling. You can't call on your feelings at will! Therefore the following practical steps should prove helpful if you are finding it difficult to forgive your spouse or others:

1. Make the decision to forgive.

This is a definite act of your will. You are empowered to forgive by the Holy Spirit, so pray for His all-powerful presence, guidance and strength. This will bring about the 'unity of forgiveness', that is, the ability for you to forgive because you yourself have been forgiven. You can

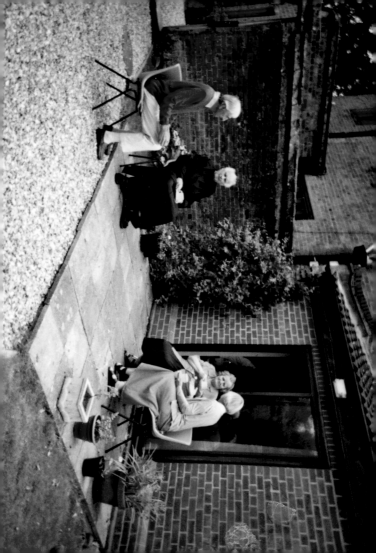

then make the commitment to God to forgive the offender.

2. Seek forgiveness yourself, for your negative thoughts and actions.

You will need to ask forgiveness from God for yourself, if necessary through the sacrament of confession, for any negative thoughts (and actions) you have had about those who have hurt you and, eventually (but *only* if appropriate and feasible), ask them to forgive you for your sinful thoughts or actions against them.

3. Make a commitment to God never to bring up the subject of the offence again.

Try to remember the person without remembering their offence. This may not be easy at first, but you need to keep recalling your commitment until it no longer holds a strong place in your memory.

4. Pray for the offender.

You cannot hold un-forgiveness and pray for a person at the same time! If the hurt persists, or you feel bitterness welling up again, you need to continue praying and, if necessary, *cry out to God for help*. In this way, the memory is eventually 'purified'.

5. Pray to God to heal your emotions and feelings.

The task of forgiving is a ceaseless struggle, but you do not battle alone! Pray to God for grace to *heal your emotions* and to harmonise them with your decision to forgive because, if you keep to your commitment to forgive, the hurts will subside in time.

2. Our Wounded Past

'You will know them by their fruits' (Matthew. 7:20)

I n this chapter we wish to explain that most of us, to a greater or lesser extent, have been wounded by various emotional problems experienced in our childhood, whether we are conscious of these or not. We will look at the effects of these wounds from the past in four specific areas, any of which are likely to result in relationship problems in the present. In each we will examine the wounding which impacts on married relationships. This should help us to recognise what is happening and thereby enable us to have some control over our responses and identify where we probably need to receive appropriate healing.

STORED MEMORIES

All childhood emotions, feelings and reactions to what our parents said or did are permanently recorded in the more primitive part of the brain, as full development is not usually reached until about seven years of age. This part of the brain cannot rationalise or differentiate between the past and present. Therefore, emotions are frequently triggered by what our spouse says or does, which is confused in our memory with similar incidents which we have experienced in our childhood. Many reactions, therefore, are archaic, inappropriate, and very destructive of married relationships. Fortunately, however, it is possible to learn to recognise these inappropriate responses and have some control over them. We will look at this in detail in the next chapter.

INNER VOWS

Inner vows usually result when having experienced, as a child, situations, actions or rejections which hurt us to such a degree that we were determined that they would not affect us again in later life. Our inner being persistently retains this self-programming, no matter what changes of mind and heart may occur in later life. This is because an inner vow resists the normal maturation process, in which we leave behind the things of childhood as we grow and mature into an adult. Inner vows resist change, and we will not grow out of them. They can become apparent when we become aware of a particular stubborn practice, or a stubborn resistance to change, or perhaps a consistent, repetitive pattern we cannot explain. When we examine these patterns in this way, although they are in our unconscious, we can often actually remember making the vow itself. Perhaps this is best shown by an example:

A medically healthy woman, married for several years, found it difficult to conceive and miscarried a number of times. Eventually, after being questioned during counselling, a memory came to mind that, when she was a young child, she was taken to see her mother's friend in a maternity ward. She was so irritated by the crying and screaming babies that, as they left, she had stamped her feet in anger and cried out: "I never want a baby; never!" *This clearly was an inner vow, a directive sent through the heart and mind to the body.* Consciously, she forgot this in later years, but her inner being did not. Now, therefore, as an adult, although she wanted to have a baby, the earlier programming was still there and functioned such that even when she conceived, she miscarried.

To break an inner vow, you will need to *repent* to the Lord for having made it and, importantly, forgive all those who may have provoked you to do so in the first place. Then you will need to *revoke* the vow or retract it in faith in Jesus' name. Finally, you will need to *replace* it fully in prayer,

expressed in several positive ways for the sake of your wounded inner child.

NEGATIVE EXPECTATIONS

Negative expectations usually result from our home environment in which, as a child, we found for example that we were constantly criticised, rejected or perhaps left out of things. This could give rise to a psychological condition in our unconscious, by which we expect a self-fulfilling prophecy to happen; in this case, to be always criticised, rejected or left out of things. By this expectancy we can unconsciously coerce or manipulate people until they do that particular thing, which then fulfils our expectation. These expectancies can have power in our life and, obviously, can cause considerable damage in adult relationships. Because they become so engrained over the years, they are difficult to recognise and overcome.

It's worth thinking in depth here; do you have any 'negative expectancies' of any kind? Do you expect to be rejected, ignored, put down or criticised? Do you find yourself saying: *"I knew that would happen"*, *"I knew he would ignore me"*, or similar comments? If you do, recognise that you have negative expectancies: every time one occurs, accept it for what it is and give it to the

Lord in prayer, asking him to heal the source. With determination and time you will find you can change the feelings as soon as you recognise them.

CHILDHOOD JUDGEMENTS

Childhood judgements occurred when we *judged our parents* or authority figures for those experiences that caused our wounding. These touch the spiritual, because they bring into action the operation of God's laws, and these cause by far the most frequent relationship problems in marriage. Let us look at some relevant laws from Scripture:

"Do not judge, and you will not be judged; because the judgements you give are the judgements you get." (Matthew 7:1-2)

"For whatever a man sows, that he will also reap." (Galatians 6:7)

"Honour your father and your mother... that it may go well with you." (Deuteronomy 5:16)

The Catechism of the Catholic Church (CCC n.2200) says: "Respecting this fourth commandment provides, along with spiritual fruits, temporal fruits of peace and prosperity. *Conversely, failure to observe it brings great harm to communities and to individuals."* This is sufficient to explain the *root* of almost every marital problem!

In every area that we judged or dishonoured our parents, whether consciously or *unconsciously*, life will not go well with us in that area; this is the outcome of the law. These judgements cause us, in our unconscious, to *'defile'* others or, as we might say, *'send out vibes'*, by character structures, habit patterns or coping mechanisms that have originated in us from our early woundings caused by these judgements. Defilement *almost* forces another person to do what we expect will happen, because laws operate as unconscious forces to influence, drive and control perceptions, attitudes and behaviour in the other person. However, we must realise that these 'vibes' can never overcome another's free will, unless it is weak or sinful.

When parents were recognisably bad or negligent, resentments are of course easily seen, admitted consciously and usually remembered well. However, when parents were 'normal and good', it is often difficult to get at the roots, because *loyalty masks reality,* both in childhood and in adult counselling. In this situation either excuses are made for the parents, or the unhelpful *"we had a very happy childhood"* comment can obscure an objective examination of the reality. It is very important to recognise at this stage that it is not a matter of *looking to blame our parents* or *finding whose fault anything was, or feeling guilty ourselves;* what is important is our *childhood reaction* to events and to what our parents said or did, and what resultant character structures were built. As a child, we may judge and react to things our parents do, whether they were good, bad or indifferent. However, law is law and it will tend to be meted back to us in those areas that we judged them. It is important to see that *what we reap is not a punishment;* it is the outcome of law.

Our childhood judgements may have been sinful, but most likely were not, considering that our age was probably below the 'age of reason', which is usually considered to be about seven years. In addition, many of these judgements would have been made *unconsciously,* and some could have even been made in our spirit whilst in our mother's womb.

As childhood judgements are so powerful in causing marital relationship problems, we will look at a number of widely different examples, to give some idea of how they have originated and their subsequent effect.

Perhaps the most difficult to discern and understand are the 'judgements' made by *babies while still in their mother's womb*. Because in some way babies feel in their spirit, at levels below reason, the hurts, fears and rejections from their parents, they react and set seeds that have to be reaped in later life. For example if the father dies, or leaves home, before the child is born, the child senses this rejection and develops a negative expectation of being abandoned or rejected in relationships in later life. Again, if the parents do not want a child and the mother finds herself pregnant, the child senses feelings of not being accepted or loved, so in later life there will be a continuous need to strive and to perform and to please, as it experiences the strong feelings of the negative expectancy of not being accepted or loved.

Consider a young baby thriving on being fed on his mother's milk, and then suddenly his mother is ill and has to discontinue feeding her baby. He is suddenly deprived and, in his spirit, may resent the substitute bottle. In his unconscious, he feels a sense of rejection, of having 'been robbed'. This resentment in later life may give rise to seemingly unexplainable, childish, self-centred behaviour in relationships, as he experiences negative expectancy of always being deprived in whatever he does.

Woundings may have resulted from over-protectiveness by parents, by the undermining of confidence, unfair treatment compared with siblings, or jealousies over the birth of a younger brother or sister. Often, shame or embarrassment of coming from a poorer family than our childhood peers, or even from having to wear 'hand-me-downs', can result in life-long difficulties in relationships.

Teasing and ridicule are very wounding experiences, and usually give rise to strong, secret judgement of the perpetrators. Sadly, *teachers* are often the authority figures that ridicule children in the classroom before their peers. These judgements, although seemingly deserved in a sense, may still be reaped in adult relationships, probably by feelings of insecurity and the need to constantly check what has been done, combined with strong denials or other defence tactics when criticised.

If you are having problems in your marriage, there is every likelihood that you and your spouse will have been wounded in some way by having made judgements on parents or authority figures in childhood. It is, therefore, important that you spend time thinking over your childhood experiences and the possible ways in which you

feel you may have been hurt or wounded as described as above.

Have you judged your parents? Remember, you are not pointing the finger at them, nor having guilt feelings yourself, but rather trying to remember how you reacted to what they said or did. Do not let your memories of a 'happy childhood', or your loyalty to your parents, obscure the fact that you inevitably must have judged your parents many times, because we all do! Therefore, *childhood judgements* will also inevitably affect your adult relationships.

Do you know whether you were wanted as a baby, or were you the sex your parents wanted? Did your mother suffer any trauma while carrying you? Was your birth normal or traumatic? Did one of your parents leave or die during your childhood? Did grandparents or other relations bring you up? Were you neglected or did you feel neglected when a sibling was born? Were you expected to take responsibilities too great for your age? Were you teased, ridiculed or bullied at school? Were you sent to a boarding school? Were your parents there for you? Were they able to help you in dealing with personal

worries and difficulties? Did they prepare you for sexual maturity?

These are just a few ideas to get you thinking! It is worth spending time on looking back at your childhood years, in order to be able to seek God's healing and be able to enjoy relationships as He originally intended. When you don't recognise your own childhood wounds, or those of your spouse, the relationship between you will inevitably deteriorate; so, clearly, you both need to go through the same exercise. Once the wounds are recognised, the resultant character structures, habit patterns or coping mechanisms then have to be identified by you both, as these cause the friction between you. How, then, can you be healed of these childhood wounds?

Scientists would say that when we fell in love, we unconsciously looked for someone who would help us finish our childhood, heal our childhood wounds and enable us to regain wholeness. This seems to be God's plan for emotional healing; His answer to the laws which are acting negatively against us. We have been created so that we can best accept emotional healing from someone who is similar to the one who wounded us. Therefore, we have probably been drawn in marriage to someone who was similar to our wounding parents. Clearly, we would not choose someone who was similar in this way, but romantic love deals with that problem! Those strong feelings of love apparently blinded us and suppressed our awareness of the negative traits in our beloved! We may not feel happy with that, but scientists have recently found that feelings of romantic love lead to a suppression of activity in the areas of the brain that control critical thought and assessment of other people, and also negative emotions!

So it is very likely that you married someone who has or will eventually appear to be incompatible in very specific ways, because that is the kind of person you need for healing. You no doubt experienced that, as your marriage progressed and romantic love subsided, you saw your spouse as he or she really is, and that is when you started to grind against one another's habit patterns. At that stage, you are likely to fear that you have made the wrong decision about your spouse, and may even think about breaking up. Alternatively, you may withdraw from the pain and set up defensive walls to protect yourself. However, in reality this is the time you should realise that, in fact, you are married to the very person who could be the most powerful healer for you, the one who could identify your

habit patterns and help and encourage you to overcome them. As you and your spouse stretch to heal each other, you both become more whole in the process.

However, you must realise that *only God can heal the original wounding.* Childhood judgements are normally not healed until you invite Jesus to accomplish this specific task. You need to take your judgements to the Cross, forgive in faith the ones who wounded you, and ask forgiveness in faith from the Lord, and through the Lord, from the ones whom you judged. You must realise that these are decisions in faith, and you may not now feel resentment against your parent or parents; however, where reaping is, judgement was the sowing, no matter how your mind or feelings may protest. The reverse, of course, may be true, in that you find it difficult or even impossible to forgive your parents. In this case you may well need help in being led through forgiveness by praying for the grace to forgive, or even the grace to be willing to forgive and recognising that this initially involves a decision and not your feelings. Seeking inner healing prayer for the 'wounded child within', from an approved Catholic healing ministry, could be very beneficial at this stage and may help you to unearth other wounds. Care needs to be taken, however, to ensure that this is a truly Catholic ministry, preferably with a priest actively involved. When it is discerned that you are ready, you will need to seek the sacrament of Confession, to receive the love of God who reconciles, and gives you that peace of mind.

You may find it useful to write a letter to your parent/s describing how you felt when you were hurt by their words, actions or omissions, expressing your forgiveness, and mentioning that you can understand the reasons why you feel they acted the way they did. This could have been due to their own wounds, their doing the best they knew how, their disciplining, their misunderstandings, or very likely it could have been your misunderstandings of what they did or did not do. This letter is *not* to give to your parent/s, even if the are still living, rather it is a therapeutic tool, and a way of bringing buried feelings and understanding to your conscious mind. Burning the letter is a very powerful symbolic gesture of finally putting the matter to rest. It may also be useful to write an imagined reply from your parent, as this really helps to bring to the surface what you may be reluctant to hear, enabling you to face the matter and truly make that decision to forgive.

You are unlikely to feel different when your wounds have been healed *but, in faith, you must believe they have been*. Once taken to the Cross, they *have* been dealt with. Unfortunately, habit patterns and character structures often keep flaring up after healing and you, or your spouse, will tend to trigger them, feed them and give them energy! We can liken the situation to a grandfather clock, where the healing has broken the mainspring of pain, but the pendulum takes much longer to stop swinging. Each habit pattern we feed pushes the pendulum. We will not be fully healed until the pendulum of the clock comes to complete rest. Your habit patterns need to be identified and isolated with the help of your spouse, and then you need to work on overcoming them with prayer and will-power. Working on one at a time, rather than all of them at once, is more likely to be successful, and quicker in the long term! Once these habit patterns no longer control your responses, your healing is complete and you can look to greatly improved relationships, especially with your spouse.

If you become aware of serious wounding in the past, such as *physical or sexual abuse*, or this comes to light through other inner healing prayer as described above, you will certainly need to find professional help; to obtain this, contact the GOODNEWS office (Catholic Charismatic Renewal Centre) England.

Telephone: (020) 7352 5298 Email: ccruk@onetel.com

Suggested further reading:

John & Paula Sandford. *The Transformation of the Inner Man.* (Tulas, Oklahoma).

Victory House Inc. 1982.

3. Confused Emotions

*'Put aside your old self... so you can put
on the new self...' (Ephesians.4:22 & 24)*

THE BRAIN AND OUR EMOTIONS

In our early life, all our childhood emotional
reactions and feelings concerning what happened
and what our parents said or did are permanently
recorded in the more primitive part of our brain. The
first five years of our life are particularly important in
this respect. At this age our brain is not fully developed
and does not become so until we are about seven years
of age. This part of the brain cannot rationalise or
differentiate between the past and present. So, one of
the most important aspects of our human experience is
to understand how brain physiology affects our
intimate, committed relationships. This helps us to
make sense out of what is often both distressing and
confusing in our relationships, the more so in a
relationship as close as our marriage.

According to neurologists, and based on the evolution of the brain, we could say we have three brains and not just one: the *Hind-brain*, which controls our automatic functions, the *Mid-brain*, which controls our emotions and instincts, and the *New brain*, which is the conscious, intentional, rational and thinking brain. This is a useful hypothesis, enabling us to understand in a simple way where our emotions are coming from.

The Mid-brain enables us to experience a very wide and rich range of emotions while we are engaged in life, but over which we have little or no control. Importantly, we need to understand and *believe* that these emotions are not controlled by the conscious part of our brain. Do we think of this when we promise to love our spouse till death parts us? We certainly can't promise to *feel* loving for a lifetime! This is why the important actions in our life ought to be the result of conscious decisions. However, we clearly need to learn to manage and understand our emotions, and learn from them, but we certainly cannot control them directly. As we develop, our emotions (rightly or wrongly) usually form the basic blueprint for thinking, acting and decision-making. They are the 'energy that moves us'. Without emotion, nothing seems really to matter; with emotion, anything can matter! However, it must be said again that, in the most important areas of our life, our actions, more profitably, need to be initiated by decisions rather than emotions.

In the emotional system, everything is either 'agreeable' or 'disagreeable', and the Mid-brain tells us that survival depends on our avoidance of pain, and repetition of pleasure. It gives rise to the tendency of *'feeling'* being somehow more important than *'thinking'*; because of this there is a common danger here, as our lowly Mid-brain, instead of the more advanced New brain, tends therefore to be the seat of our value judgements. In other words, it is likely to decide whether our New brain has a 'good' idea or not, by whether it *feels* true and right! The advanced New brain should, ideally, control our lives and our marriages but, unfortunately, that rarely seems to happen in the real world. Most marriages, sadly, tend to run on Hind- and Mid-brain energy; that is, the more primitive part!

Our emotions reside within us; that is, they are 'stored' in our Mid-brain, and they are constantly being triggered by stimuli from outside us. In our marriage this is most likely to be our spouse! Therefore, we need to recognise that the Mid-brain has a limited and primitive impression of the outside world, and constantly confuses people and events!

Often, for example in our marriage, the Mid-brain will tend to confuse our spouse with our parent! Although our rational and intelligent New brain clearly knows the difference between our spouse and our parent, the Mid-brain, which triggers and controls our emotions, reactions, and protective impulses, constantly *mixes them up!* Therefore, if our spouse criticizes us and we have a history of a critical parent or teacher, our Mid-brain may react emotionally as though we were once again living with, and dealing with, that old critic. This happens even when we consciously know that our spouse is different from the old critic and that we are now, of course, an adult and not a child. This is also the reason why we can often experience intense feelings in our marriage with our spouse; for example, fear or helplessness, although rationally we know there is no need to fear or feel helpless.

When something happens in the present that is similar to something that happened years ago in childhood, the Mid-brain connects the present experience to the old experience, without recognising the 'old' as 'old'. This is because it lives in the 'eternal now', having no concept of time. The emotion that was experienced as a child is brought into the present situation and the combined emotion, of then and now, is experienced. *So nearly all of the upset, hurt, emotion and reactions we experience in our marriage are, most likely, archaic and related to our early childhood history.* Very little, if any, is related to the present event.

Much of the intense emotion that arises in relationships is because the Mid-brain treats emotional risk as a survival issue, and mixes the past with the present, confusing people, events and time. It jumps into action and tries to make us take 'evasive action' by hiding, fighting, running, 'freezing', or submitting. We may *hide* by lying, keeping secrets, burying ourselves in the television, or not sharing. We may *fight* by arguing, shouting, blaming or criticising. We may *run* by leaving the house, going for a drive or working late. We may *'freeze'* by saying or doing nothing, or we may *submit* by giving in or accepting abuse. We need to recognise these evasive actions, which indicate we *are not feeling safe with each other*; more importantly, we must believe that these are mostly not rational reactions, but are archaic and from the past!

Having understood how our brain works, we can see that *nobody can cause, or be responsible for, our emotions*; these lie within us, stored in our Mid-brain, and may be stimulated by others, but the responsibility of expressing these is ours alone. If we can analyse where they come from they can become a learning experience and lead to our growth.

If you have experienced any intense emotions, like fear, helplessness, terror, embarrassment, or put-downs, for no readily apparent reason when you have been with your spouse, or you have responded inappropriately with a 'knee-jerk' response and then wondered what made you say that, you will now, no doubt, understand what has been happening. This knowledge itself, in time, will help you to gain some control over your reactions, and help you to make them more appropriate and Christian. However, you really need a more practical and easier way of helping you to recognize these connections between your Mid-brain and the present, which are causing you these problems - a tool to relate these past emotional reactions that are in your unconscious to your present experiences and behaviour.

TRANSACTIONAL ANALYSIS

Transactional Analysis (T.A.) is such a tool, because it shows you how to recognize, in a conversation (a transaction), when a person is coming from their unconscious past. You are able to do this from their words, attitudes and actions. It will not take you long to learn and recognize these signs! However, you will perhaps

need more explanations and examples to make this easier.

We know now that every event in our life, and the emotional reaction to it, are recorded in our Mid-brain, and that the first five years of our life are uniquely important in this respect. These events (especially the feelings associated with them) are constantly being replayed when triggered by some external stimulus, and mostly remain in our unconscious.

T.A. is a way of relating these past emotional reactions to our present experience and behaviour. If we are willing to act against inhibiting or crippling feelings we will, with God's help, be able to change our habits of behaviour in certain situations and then the course of our life. However, it is necessary to unearth these buried feelings; firstly, we need to recognise them by observing ourselves in interaction with others in what is called a 'transaction': someone offers us a stimulus in word or gesture and we react with a response (e.g. a normal conversation). Understanding T.A. enables us to analyse the transaction and helps us to recognise and evaluate the underlying emotional influences of both stimulus and response.

T.A. begins with a supposition that all people are inflicted with feelings of inferiority from infancy - of being **'not OK'** - and most never fulfill their potential because they don't overcome this and become **'OK'**. 'OK' means we refuse to be paralysed by our faults and emotional problems, and we are determined to take control of our life by bringing our 'New brain' into action. *We need to make the choice to move from the position 'I'm not OK – You're OK" to the position 'I'm OK – You're OK'.*

To make this choice we must first recognise that we each have three ego states within us: PARENT – ADULT – CHILD. We flit from one to the other, according to how we are stimulated. We can learn to recognise these three ego states in others, and ourselves, by *analysing the attitude, the gestures and the actual words used* in our conversations with people. When we have learned to identify which ego state we are coming from, and are adept at getting in touch with it, we are then in the position to put our Adult in charge. In that case, we are controlled neither by the narrow and fixed positions of our Parent nor the insatiable needs of the Child. Our life should be governed gently but forcibly by reason - our *Adult*; but we must recognise and love the boundaries and wisdom of our *Parent* and the wonder, enthusiasm and creativity of our *Child*. We must give our Adult time to sort out our Parent and Child from reality, by counting to ten if necessary! We must work from a system of ethical values and concentrate on developing a *strong Adult*. This is the way we should react as a mature and loving Christian!

The Parent Ego State

The Parent ego state is a huge collection of recordings, in our Mid-brain, of external events seen or heard in the first five years of our life. These are recordings of the manner and pronouncements of our real parents or substitutes; they are recorded 'straight' and unquestioned, without editing, as we had no ability to do so at that age. They include all the early, non-verbal communications from our parents, such as tone of voice, facial expressions, cuddling or non-cuddling, together with all the more elaborate verbal rules and regulations directed by our parents as we became able to understand words. Included here are the thousands of 'noes' and 'don'ts' directed at the toddler. Most of these recordings will tend to be negative, as we learn, explore, experiment and test our autonomy! Later come the more complicated pronouncements, such as "If you sit in a draught you'll catch a cold", "Waste not want not", "You are judged by the friends you make", etc.

The significant point to remember is that, whether these rules or sayings are true or false, good or bad ethically, they are *recorded as truth*. It is a permanent recording and cannot be erased, and is available for replay throughout life. When we are acting in the Parent ego state, our behaviour is determined by these messages, which are fixed, unchanging, and dogmatic. They are, for the most part, authoritative, critical, restricting, controlling and inhibiting. We use words and phrases such as 'should', 'shouldn't', 'always', 'never', 'once and for all', 'if I were you', 'nonsense', 'how many times have I told you?'

A typical Parent-to-Parent transaction: *"It's ridiculous Jane wearing make-up at her age; I'm going to stop this once and for all."*

"Yes, we've got to nip this in the bud before it's too late."

The Child Ego State

The Child ego state is a recording of all the *internal events*: that is, the responses to what we saw and heard, and what we 'felt' and understood, while the external events were being recorded in our Parent. All our emotional reactions, from ecstasy to despair, are stored here in the Mid-brain, as also are all the hurts we acquired in our early relationships.

When we are acting from the Child ego state, we are spontaneous, lively, creative, and motivated by feelings. We will tend to be primitive and self-depreciating, but can also be capable of excitement, wonder and enthusiasm. Our behaviour shows such expressions as tears, quivering lips, pouting, whining, temper tantrums, downcast eyes, sobbing, giggling, squirming, shrieking, etc., and we use expressions such as 'I want', 'I need', 'I wish', 'I guess', 'I don't care', 'I don't know', 'I feel', 'I'm going to', and 'Give me', etc. We are, however, also acting from our Child ego state when we are creative, artistic, and fun-loving.

A typical Child-to-Child transaction, between husband and wife: *"Whether you like it or not, I'm going to that concert tomorrow night."*

"I don't care what you do; I'm going to the pub anyway, with the lads."

The Adult Ego State

The Adult ego state develops as soon as we begin to do things from our own awareness and original thought; this self-actualisation continues to be fed from exploring and testing. We begin to be able to tell the difference between life as it was taught and demonstrated to us (Parent), life as we felt it or wished it (Child), and life as we now figure it out ourselves (Adult).

The New brain computes information from three sources: the Parent, the Child, and the data the Adult has already gathered and is gathering. The important function of the Adult in us is to *listen to, review, and evaluate the fixed parental messages that were recorded as 'the truth' in the Mid-brain, to re-evaluate them, and decide what to act upon and what to act against.* The Adult also listens to the emotional hurts and enthusiasms of the Child, and allows or disallows the Child's whims in the light of mature values and rational decisions.

When we are acting from the Adult ego state, we use words such as 'why', 'what', 'where', 'when', 'who', and 'how', and also 'how much', 'in what way', 'true', 'false', 'probable', 'possible', 'I think', 'I see', 'it is my opinion', etc. These all indicate data processing.

A typical Adult-to-Adult transaction between husband and wife:

"I think it would probably be a good time to spray the roses this evening."

"Yes, I agree, because the wind has died down at last, and they forecast a dry spell."

'Knee-Jerk Responses'

'Knee-Jerk Responses' can be a problem in relationships, especially in our marriage, causing or resulting from one of us coming from the Parent ego state and the other from the Child ego state. We tend to *trigger off* a response from the opposite ego state; that is, the *Child is likely to trigger off a Parent response*. For example:

"Why is it always me who has to put the bin out every week?"(Whining Child)

"You poor thing! Not complaining again! You ought to be helping me with the washing-up, too!" (Parent)

Similarly, the *Parent is likely to trigger off a Child response;* for example:

"You never keep the spare room tidy; it's an absolute mess!" (Parent)

"So what?! Half the stuff is yours anyway!" (Aggressive Child)

Or:

"Sorry dear, I'll go up and tidy it now." (Submissive Child)

In both these examples the conversations are *between a wife and a husband!*

In your marriage you need to be particularly aware of these *'knee-jerk reaction'* transactions, as they are likely to be the source of many resentments, arguments and quarrels. You can quickly recognise when your spouse is coming from their Parent, by the strong *'gut feeling'* you experience within yourself as you feel you are being talked down to, or they are being inappropriately authoritative or demanding. These provoke archaic responses from your Child, which may be aggressive or submissive, as shown above, either of which is going to be harmful to your married relationship. If your spouse is coming from their Child, you will probably be irritated, annoyed, or angry, which will provoke a Parent response from you, which again will be archaic and inappropriate. If you find you are being 'triggered off' in either of these ways, the answer is to give an Adult response, which will usually bring the other to

their Adult ego state (eventually), because it brings the rational New brain into action. It may be a good idea to agree a *codeword* like 'Ouch!' to bring to the attention of your spouse that they are coming over from an inappropriate ego state! You need, however, to be very careful here, as a remark like *"There you go again, coming from your Parent"* is certainly unlikely to go down well!

If you are to grow in maturity in your married life together and become *'OK'*, you need to learn to come from your Adult, or approve your Parent or Child through your Adult, if you deem it appropriate. As St. Paul puts it: *"You must give up your old way of life; you must put aside your old self, which gets corrupted by following illusory desires. Your mind must be renewed by a spiritual revolution so that you can put on the new self that has been created in God's way, in the goodness and holiness of the truth."* (Ephesians. 4:22-24)

Now we have explained about these ego states and how, by words and attitudes, you can identify what is happening when you communicate with your spouse, you will soon recognise who's coming from where! This will enable you quite quickly to develop the practice of coming from your Adult, which at the same time helps your spouse to do the same. **If this has been a problem in your marriage, you will be surprised how quickly things can improve dramatically, if even only one of you works at it!**

Suggested further reading:

Thomas Harris. *I'm OK – You're OK* (London. Pan Books. 1982.)

John Powell S.J. *The Secret of Staying in Love* (California. Tabor Publishing.1974.)

4. Communication

'Be quick to listen but slow to speak.' (James 1:19)

INTRODUCTION

Communication is a technical skill that must come as a result of a decision. Good communication is essential if there is to be a growing trust and closeness between a husband and wife. It is the *very vehicle of relationship*. It is the pathway between two minds and an essential ingredient of 'the two becoming one'. No relationship, of course, can exist without some kind of communication, even if it is not verbal; and many consider lack of communication to be the primary reason for relationships breaking down. It is true, of course, that failure to communicate is almost always involved in relationship breakdown, but it is more the *instrument of breakdown* rather than the cause.

There are two major types of verbal communication, each of which has its own objective;

these are *Discussion* and *Dialoguing*. We will briefly describe them.

DISCUSSION

Discussion is used to inform our spouse about our thoughts, plans, opinions, etc.; that is, basically, sharing things of a predominantly intellectual nature, and this does not make us vulnerable. It enables us to show our spouse where we are coming from and our views on various topics; also it enables us to make plans and decisions and to exchange ideas together. This includes, of course, much of our 'everyday conversations' on priorities, jobs, plans, observations, comments and anecdotes.

DIALOGUING

Dialoguing involves matters of the heart; that is, the sharing of our feelings and emotions with our spouse. This is vitally important, as breakdown in human love is always due to emotional problems. We need to have the emotional clearance and ventilation that dialogue brings. We need continuous support of our personal worth in our love-relationship and, when we are deprived of this, we can get feelings of fundamental failure. Dialoguing - the sharing of our emotions - gives release and perspective, and enables us to come to a deeper knowledge, understanding and fuller acceptance of each other in love. Dialogue is based on the assumption that feelings and emotions are *natural reactions, which have no moral implications.* We do not have to explain, excuse, or give reasons; it's OK to feel what we feel. The danger lies in ignoring, denying, or refusing to report our feelings. There is no place for argument in dialogue, as it is essentially an exchange of feelings. It must not be manipulative, nor must it be judgmental of our spouse or of our self.

The true disposition to dialogue is that you *want your spouse to know you as you really are.* When you marry, you marry a virtual stranger! How ever long your courtship, you will, in all likelihood, know very little of the real person you are marrying. Lives are so often occupied by projecting on others – our parents, our teachers, our employers, and our friends – an image of ourselves which we think they will like. Therefore, you can end up marrying, in part, an image! An exciting aspect of marriage, indeed, should be the discovery of the real person you have married, and loving them as they really are, warts and all! Therefore, you should constantly use dialogue to exchange your mutual understanding, not in pursuit of any victory. You

want your spouse to share your most precious possession - *yourself!*

The other side of dialogue is, of course, listening with empathy; active listening, to hear what our spouse is *feeling*; to honestly say "I hear you, I am sharing your feeling, I am feeling it with you." As a true listener in dialogue, we acknowledge and respect the otherness of the speaker, offer no solutions, suggestions or unnecessary interruptions, and always remember that underlying truth: feelings are OK.

If your spouse is uncooperative, you should ask yourself a few questions about how you have approached the dialogue yourself; your motivation, your response, your listening, and any other action or reaction which may have caused your spouse to lose trust. In your love-relationship, if you truly open up to your spouse as an act of self-disclosure, you will usually find this will be reciprocated.

Expressing your feelings and emotions by writing dialogue letters to your spouse, instead of voicing them, is very powerful and rewarding. It helps you to get in touch with your unconscious more readily than when you search for words to express yourself. As an exercise to grow in

intimacy, we suggest you dialogue weekly; that is, write about your feelings and emotions, (not your thoughts, ideas or solutions) on a particular topic that is important to you. Both you and your spouse must select the same topic! Then pray for the Holy Spirit to guide you and give you the words to write. Each of you goes to a separate room to write, so as not to put your spouse off by seeing you writing! Then, in the form of a letter to your spouse, write spontaneously for ten minutes without stopping, about the feelings and emotions which come to mind when you consider that particular topic. Try to fill one side of an A4 sheet of paper. If you cannot think of anything to say, it is best to just start writing *anything* that occurs to you; then you will find your unconscious will do the rest, rather like priming a pump! Don't worry about grammar or punctuation, just keep writing; this is not an English test! After ten minutes or so, come together and exchange your letters or read them out. Then share your further thoughts and feelings in *love*. This is really the only way to grow in intimacy, and you will find the exercise, if done regularly, will enrich and strengthen your marriage.

CONFLICT

Conflict will occur in all marriages and must be expected and accepted. Differences should be accepted; conflicts need to be recognised and resolved correctly and satisfactorily. Things that one spouse dislikes in the other may have to be brought into the open by confrontation in order to resolve the conflict that is there. Sadly, couples often allow themselves to get involved in negative patterns when dealing with conflict. There appear to be four major forms of negative conflict resolutions:

Escalation

Escalation occurs when spouses respond back and forth increasingly negatively with damaging verbal abuse.

It is imperative to learn to recognise escalation as soon as it starts in order to short-circuit it before any real damage occurs. Softening your tone and acknowledging your spouse's point of view are powerful steps in helping to defuse the tension and thereby end escalation.

Painful Put-downs

Painful put-downs result when one spouse subtly or caustically puts the other down.

To prevent these you must acknowledge and show respect for each other's viewpoint, respect for each other's character, and an emphasis on building-up. This leads to intimacy and reduces anger and resentment.

Withdrawals and Avoidance

Withdrawals and avoidance are similar, but different, patterns in which one spouse shows an unwillingness to get into or stay with an important discussion that needs to be talked through.

If you recognise this pattern in your marriage, you must first realise that you are not independent of one another. Your actions cause reactions, and vice-versa. Therefore, you need to work together to change or prevent this kind of negative pattern. Pursuers must back off and pursue more constructively, and withdrawers must deal more directly with the issues in hand.

Negative Interpretations

Negative interpretations occur when one spouse consistently believes that the motives of the other are far more negative than is really the case.

It is extremely difficult to overcome this pattern of negative interpretation, as only the one who has adopted this pattern can control how they interpret their spouse's behaviour. Possible helps might be: firstly, to examine whether they are over-emphasising the negative interpretations of their partner's behaviour; secondly, to push themselves to look for evidence that is contrary to their interpretation; thirdly, to look honestly at whether there might be personal reasons for maintaining their negative interpretations, such as seeing themselves as a kind of martyr, or perhaps a need to be seen as the one who truly cares for the partnership.

However, these honest self-reflections are always very difficult. You need to learn to accept each other in love, and concentrate on seeing each other positively.

Clearly, if you are both constantly involved in any of these very hurtful conflict patterns you will both need the graces of regular sacramental

Confession to enable you to demonstrate practically to one another your true and honest intention to tackle the suggestions given. When you fail, immediately seek reconciliation between yourselves by asking and giving forgiveness.

When we see the damage caused by any of these four negative conflict-management patterns, we will recognise how imperative it is that conflict- and problem-solving are approached in more *constructive* ways. For example, employing tools that enable us to hear each other, and thus obviating the likelihood of any of these described destructive patterns occurring. However, before we use tools, we will need to adopt a *correct approach and right attitude* towards conflict and confrontation, to help us to be gracious and to see our spouse in a positive and loving light. As St. Paul in his letter to the Ephesians says:

"…Get rid of all bitterness, rage and anger, brawling and slander, along with every form of malice. Be kind and compassionate to one another, forgiving each other, just as in Christ God forgave you." Ephesians 4:29-32.

Conflicts have a knack of cropping up at times when you are least able to deal with them; perhaps just as you are off to work, or perhaps

when you are just home after a heavy shopping session! So often you can make the great mistake of trying to deal with them there and then. You are probably very tired, irritable, desperate for a rest, or perhaps anxious to get to work on time as you are a bit late... whatever the situation, you are certainly not in the best mode to be rational, considerate or understanding to your spouse. It is far better to acknowledge that you have a disagreement, and suggest talking it out at a mutually agreeable time (preferably) later that day. It is, however, imperative that you both *keep to this agreement*, however reluctant you may be to pick up the subject again! If you do not deal with it then, it will most certainly crop up again. When selecting a time for dealing with the conflict, you should be sensitive to your own and to your spouse's mood, tiredness, busyness, and health.

Acceptance of your spouse is very important when disagreement is raging as, so often, there is a distortion of vision. True unconditional love helps you to accept your spouse as they are, and accept that they have a right to have a different opinion; this helps you to see the situation as it really is. Acceptance also encourages you to *listen* to what your spouse is *really* saying, and not half-listen and consequently 'get hold of the wrong end of the stick', as it is so easy to do.

CONFRONTATION

There are bound to be occasions, situations and even regular occurrences when we need to confront our spouse, because we feel that what is being done or spoken is unacceptable to us. However, we need to be certain that confrontation is necessary. Perhaps we should try 'confronting' ourselves first! For example: Why is this behaviour or situation bothering us? Are we being just plain selfish? Is our perception warped, bent or biased? Are we hypersensitive, insecure or paranoid? Or are we narrow-minded, short-sighted, prejudiced, or even bigoted? Could it be that we are opinionated, hypercritical, or fussy? Are we being doctrinaire, dogmatic, pedantic or snobbish, over-zealous, fanatical or perfectionist?

You still need to decide (test) whether confrontation is required. Ask yourself: *"Is confrontation on this matter good for our marriage?"* and *"is it good for my spouse?"* It needs to be both and, if it is, then see it as your duty to challenge your spouse's attitude or behaviour as an act of love. Because confrontation is bringing up conflict in order to solve a problem, you need to

be extra sensitive, and we suggest you use the helpful hints below.

In confrontation it is important to communicate *the feelings you experience* when your spouse does whatever is causing the conflict with you. These messages should try to express *underlying feelings* like hurt, disappointment, or helplessness, rather than the less helpful surface feelings like anger or hatred. By giving a *personal statement* you are telling your spouse how you feel and why you feel it, and you are *not* blaming or criticising. You both need to remember that feelings are OK, and you should not be blamed or criticised for expressing them! So, when confronting, you need to make it clear what *you are feeling* when your spouse does something you do not like, and *why* you feel this way; this is called an *'I'-message,* for obvious reasons!

For example:

- "*I feel weary* when I find your clothes on the bedroom floor, because I seem to spend so much time tidying the room."

- *"I feel quite distant from you* when you spend so much time working on your laptop, because I feel I'm not important to you."

It will be seen that these 'I-messages' all have the same basic structure, which makes it useful for remembering and for practising:

"I feel......... when......... because........."

It is very important, however, to note that the following statements: "I feel *that you…*" or *"*I think *that you…"* are **not** 'I'-messages expressing *feelings* but are, in fact, stating *opinions, criticisms or judgements,* of your spouse. These should be avoided at all costs in confrontation.

For confrontation to be effective and loving it is necessary to separate behaviour from character, to separate 'the sin from the sinner'; that is, the spouse's behaviour, and not the spouse's character, is confronted. In addition, even when using 'I'-messages, there is a need to choose carefully the words used, as it is so easy to phrase confrontation with words which will trigger one of the negative patterns we looked at above.

SAFE AND CLEAR COMMUNICATION

To handle a conflict well is critical for the future of a marriage, so we need to be able to communicate clearly and safely. This requires using agreed strategies and techniques that add structure and rules to our interactions, and help to keep them cool. The **Speaker-Listener** technique, developed by Drs Markman and Scott, is designed primarily for dealing with sensitive issues or volatile subjects, enabling each spouse to hear clearly what the other is actually saying, thus ensuring that the subject to be aired is discussed fully. This is essential before problem-solving is attempted. The technique needs to be practised initially on easy topics, so that the couple can get familiar with it before they need to use it!

The person who starts the discussion is the **Speaker**, the one who holds the floor, and it is a good idea to have some sort of object (e.g. a small book, or coaster, etc.) to represent the floor. The spouse without the floor is the **Listener**. The Speaker presents his or her feelings and concerns and the Listener listens and paraphrases, until the floor is passed to the Listener, who then becomes the Speaker, and the roles are reversed. This can be done any number of times, until the subject is talked out; it is important, however, **not** to try problem-solving at this stage. It is also important to keep to the same subject and not to become sidetracked onto other issues. The flow can be stopped for clarification of something said, or if the rules are not being adhered to. It may be useful to agree a signal beforehand, to stop things if one or other feels that things are getting out of hand.

The Speaker should talk in sentences short enough that the listener can remember and paraphrase; if this paraphrase is not quite accurate, the Speaker should politely repeat what they said to the Listener. The issue should be presented using 'I'-statements, talking about their side of the issue, their feelings, emotions and concerns. The floor can be passed to the Listener at any time to hear their side of the issue.

The Listener should paraphrase what the Speaker is saying, repeating back in their own words what the Speaker conveyed, but should not include their own thoughts or anything said at any other time. Explanations or examples may be requested of the Speaker, but paraphrasing should be the norm. It is essential (but may in practice be very difficult) not to comment or express an opinion as a Listener, and that includes facial expressions and body language! The Listener must try to concentrate on what the Speaker is communicating, and not start mentally preparing their response; they should also concentrate on showing respect for their spouse's point of view, even if it is not agreed with.

The Speaker-Listener technique allows issues to be fully aired and explored. It helps to keep the interchange cool, and should ensure that both parties have heard and understood what the other has said, thus counteracting the destructive patterns of dealing with conflict outlined above. The scene is thus set for solving the problems involved with the issue. In many instances, and researchers tell us in something like *70 percent* of cases, after an excellent discussion, there's really no problem-solving to be done! Having a good discussion was enough. It seems that what spouses want most when they are upset is not necessarily agreement, or even change, but just *to feel heard and understood.*

However, there will be times when the 'Speaker-Listener' discussions of problems or issues will naturally lead to the next step: of working together to *find specific solutions to the problems.* There are a number of well-known techniques for problem-solving which can be used, such as "brainstorming" and "force field analysis".

Suggested further reading:

Fighting for Your Marriage Howard Markham, Scott Stanley & Susan Blumberg. (San Francisco. Jossey-Bass Publishers. 1994.)

5. Priorities In Family Life

'Love your neighbour as yourself' *(Mt.22:39)*

We need to ask ourselves where our priorities lie in our family life and, more importantly, whether we are observing these priorities, which are clearly laid down for us in Holy Scripture. If we are not, all our relationships will be likely to suffer in consequence. We can easily believe we are giving priority to one relationship and be oblivious to the fact that we are giving less, or very little, priority to another. Unfortunately, too, our priorities are often misdirected without our being aware of this until our relationships suffer. However, we must stress that we are talking here about priorities; that is, our normal mode of operation, our normal way of doing things. Priorities are not cast-iron rules and they may have to be changed from time to time for special or routine purposes, or circumvented for emergencies, but only on a temporary basis. So, what are our priorities then? We are told in Matthew's Gospel that Jesus says: *"You must love the Lord your God with all your heart, with all your soul and with all your mind. This is the greatest and first commandment. The second resembles it: You must love your neighbour as yourself."* (Matthew 22:37-39).

FIRST PRIORITY

From Holy Scripture, then, we can clearly state that our first priority must be our *personal relationship with God.* What do we mean by this in our married life?

Is your first priority your relationship with God? As a Christian you need to start each day with a fundamental decision that you are going to live by the power of the Holy Spirit, and not by the power of your own human nature; you should allow the Holy Spirit to change your way of thinking, in essence to put on the mind of Christ. By reading God's word in Holy Scripture, you could discern God's will for you each day. Then if you start each day with your spouse in prayer, committing your lives to Jesus and seeking God's wisdom and revelation for you both, you will be able to fix your thoughts on God and on how much He loves you, and you will find you can love and forgive others and reach out to those in need. You need to check constantly whether you are living the 'new life', throughout the day. If you are, you should experience peace, joy, love

and the other fruits of the Spirit. If you are not, you will see anger, frustration, turmoil and division. If you experience these, you need to repent and recommit yourselves to the Spirit. (See also *Prayer* and *Forgiveness* in Chapter 1.) If you truly put God first in your marriage you will be blessed and enabled to minister daily to your spouse and bring Christ into your relationship in a very real way. Remember that God is the third person in your marriage!

SECOND PRIORITY

After God, we are told, we must love our neighbour as *our self*. This implies that, before we love our neighbour, we must first love ourselves; in fact, we are unable to love anyone else without loving ourselves first. Psychologists tell us that *all* psychological problems, from the slightest neuroses to the deepest psychoses, are symptomatic of the frustration of our fundamental human need for a sense of personal worth, self-love, or self-esteem. Psychologists also tell us that our self-image is the radical determining factor of our behaviour. Therefore, true and realistic self-esteem is the basic element in the health of our personality. We act and relate to other people in accordance with the way we think of and feel about ourselves. How do we love ourselves? Firstly we must be convinced that we *should* love ourselves. True self-love, self-acceptance, or self-esteem, is not egoism, vanity, conceit or narcissism. We should recognize that we are born unique and of great giftedness. We are mysterious and unrepeatable in the whole course of human history and, importantly, we are made after the image and likeness of God Himself, with a unique role to play in God's creation!

Dr Debbie Cherry, in her book *Child-proofing Your Marriage*, suggests some steps to help build up your self-esteem, so that you can reach out to love your spouse, having established a healthy self-love yourself. You should learn to use positive self-talk, by complimenting and affirming yourself as a lovable, worthwhile, valuable person, because God says you are. You are, after all, God's work of art! You need to forgive yourself, and stop living in the past and reliving your mistakes, because God has forgiven you. In all humility you should celebrate your strengths, successes and talents. Always accept compliments and do this with a "thank you" and a smile; if appropriate, give the credit to God, and never contradict in false modesty. Set realistic goals, in order to set yourself up for success by achieving them. Stop comparing yourself to others - you are no judge of yourself

or others! Associate with encouragers, by being surrounded by supportive and positive people.

THIRD PRIORITY

The command *to love our neighbour* must begin with our nearest neighbour - our *family*. Within our family, if we are married, clearly the priority must be to our *spouse*. By reading Chapter 5 of St. Paul's Letter to the Ephesians, we should be in no doubt as to our wife or husband being our priority relationship as our neighbour, and also be in no doubt as to how God is calling us to love our spouse. In fact, this relationship between husband and wife is the highest relationship between humans spoken of in the Bible. It is the only relationship where God said: *"The two shall become one"*. This is not two halves that make one whole, but two whole persons forming an entirely new whole; that is, *"becoming one flesh"*.

Leaving

In Genesis it says: *"...a man leaves his father and mother and joins himself to his wife..."*(Gen. 2:24). Older translations often used the word 'cleaves' for 'joins', which expresses perhaps a stronger reality, almost suggesting gluing together, with the further implication of the damage done to *both* when separated. Only the 'man' is mentioned here because, in that time and in that culture, the wife was the one that moved to the husband's home. *Leaving is an important aspect of giving our spouse priority.* Leaving must be clean and clear-cut; just as a baby cannot grow up unless the umbilical cord is cut, so marriage cannot grow and develop as long as no real leaving, or clear separation from one's family has taken place. If young couples have no chance to start their own home completely separate from their families, there is a grave danger that the in-laws will interfere continuously; this may be for the best of intentions or not, but the result may be the same! Leaving creates a breathing space in which the love between parents and children can grow and prosper. *The extended family can only function successfully if the nuclear family is intact and healthily independent.* If we have not fully made the break with our own parents, we will have difficulty in adjusting to our in-laws!

If you feel this relates to you, and you recognize problems that have arisen due to any of the reasons above, you need to sit down with your spouse and gently and lovingly look at how you can improve the situation. It may even be necessary to talk with your parents and/or in-laws, again lovingly and gently!

Your full commitment in marriage has to be to your spouse. So often your parents can become a haven to which you may return when the going gets difficult. This is contrary to God's law. In misplacing these priorities, the situation is doomed to bring increasing troubles to you both, over and above what you are trying to leave. You must refocus your lives on *each other* and remember your duty is to minister to one another in love, and to live your sacrament daily.

If you have very close relationships with the other members of your family, or in-laws, especially your brothers and sisters and your brothers and sisters-in-law, these have to take a lesser priority now you are married, in order that you may devote your attention and energies to your spouse. This is not easy and, if you have not stepped back from these relationships already, it will be even more difficult when you do. Leaving is usually not joyful, and you will experience pain in many of your relationships and perhaps you may even shed many tears, but remember: *leaving is the price of happiness* with your spouse. Leaving also means giving a *lesser* priority to all those things that, prior to your marriage, meant so much to you and occupied so much of your time: maybe your business, your career, your hobbies, your talents, your interests, your sports, your house, your church, or your friends. All of these have to be put into a *proper perspective*, but not neglected, if you wish to develop the thrilling oneness of relationship that God intended you to enjoy as a couple.

Having established that your spouse comes second only to God in your life, and you have satisfactorily put all those other areas of your life into proper perspective, you must obviously endeavour to *maintain this equilibrium* in order to live your sacrament daily. You must be aware of the encroachment of relations and friends (in the flesh or on your mobile!), attitudes, and activities such as TV, browsing the Internet, etc., which may subtly become priorities in your life to the detriment of your spouse and, inevitably, your marriage.

Work

Work can, perhaps, be a great danger in confusing our priorities. Excessive overtime, working at the weekends, bringing work home, pursuing the relentless desire for promotion and climbing to the top; and all this, perhaps, being done genuinely for the benefit of our spouse and family - *but at what cost to our relationship?*

Work is a problem area that almost seems inevitable in the western culture in which we live. When we get married these days, we want a home of our own; and raising a mortgage to buy one seems to be the only answer in most cases, as property to rent is frequently not available. To pay the deposit and to furnish the property usually means we both need to work for an adequate income. This also means that we only have the evenings and weekends to 'live and enjoy' our marriage, and this is also usually the only time we have for housework, gardening, DIY, etc. This is not good news for us as a newly-married couple! Two or three years later, a baby may be on the way; the wife gives up her job, the income drops and our expenses are going to increase. The husband maybe tries to supplement his income by working extra hours or taking on an extra job; this produces more stress and less or no quality time for us to be together, and the focus inevitably turns to the baby and all of its needs. This is an all-too-common scenario, to which there is no easy answer.

If this is your story, what can you do? To save your marriage it is essential that the correct priorities are in some way made concrete in your

relationship, as a matter of some urgency. You both need to discuss how to achieve a more satisfactory balance of the necessary 'work time', in order to be able to enjoy some quality time together.

Quality Time Together

It cannot be stressed too much that having *quality time together* is an absolute *must* if a marriage is to survive and mature. By *quality time* is meant a time of recreation together, when you can enjoy each other by sharing of yourselves. It is *not* a time to discuss finances, children, or jobs that need to be done around the home! You may only be able to find one or two hours a week if the situation is as difficult as described above, but even this is a valuable lifeline for your marriage. Ideally, you should work towards having an evening a week for your time together, a 'couple's evening', a time when you will not be interrupted (no pets or mobile phones!). As your children grow older, this needs to be recognized by them as 'Mum & Dad's evening'; and they in turn should also be able to look forward to an evening or weekend when they can enjoy quality time *with* Mum and Dad.

So often our 'couple's time' is not planned or scheduled and, therefore, never happens; then the priorities become obscured and the job subtly takes priority over wife and children. This is not exclusive to men, of course; many career women, or women pursuing higher education, can similarly let their priorities to their husband and children suffer.

You need to be constantly on guard, and continually keep checking where your true priorities lie. To help determine the true position, you should constantly dialogue your real deep feelings with one another, and be sensitive to what you hear and ready to change what you are doing, *if* your priorities are not ordered correctly.

Children

No doubt the commonest, subtlest, and most gradual erosion of our priority to our spouse is when we give this priority instead to our *children*. This applies, perhaps, more often to the mother, but by no means exclusively so. Fathers, and often both parents, in giving loving care and attention to their children, so often *unintentionally neglect their relationship with their spouse.* This may be inevitable in the short term but, when it becomes the norm, it may even not be noticed by the couple due to the increasing role - usually for both of them - of the children in the life of the family in general, as they are brought up and educated. The constant demands by the children on time, energy and money, often result in the deterioration of the relationship between the spouses. It is, tragically, only when the children start to leave home that we realize we have little or nothing in common with our spouse, because we have slowly drifted apart over the years without being really aware of it. This is an all-too-common cause of marital disharmony. The larger the family, the more likely this is to happen, of course, as the time span is lengthened.

You need to remember that you made a commitment to your spouse *"till death parts you"*, and reflect perhaps that your children are only *'lent'* to you for a number of years. You should not forget, either, that your children *should* see your marriage relationship as *a model and a role* for their own future relationships, this being an important element of living your sacrament.

FOURTH PRIORITY

Our children must, of course, take priority over everything else, apart from God, our self and our spouse. Paul, in his Letter to Timothy, says: *"He must manage his own family well and see that his children obey him with proper respect."* (1Timothy 3:4)

In the Catechism of the Catholic Church (CCC n.2221) it says: *"The fecundity of conjugal love cannot be reduced solely to the procreation of children, but must extend to their moral education and their spiritual formation. "The **role of parents in education** is of such importance that it is almost impossible to provide an adequate substitute. The right and duty of parents to educate their children are primordial and inalienable."*

Physical begetting of children, then, is only the start of life for them; this is not complete until they learn, from us, who God is and how to love Him, and then we become *fully* parents to them.

In the context of priorities, the *duties* of the parents are the prime concern, so techniques and practical advice to help in parenting are not dealt with here. However, these matters are obviously intimately associated with the marriage relationship and our relationship with our children, and can cause ongoing problems between spouses.

If you are experiencing serious problems in this area, which are being reflected in a deterioration of your relationship with your

spouse, you should seek professional help, as this is beyond the scope of this guide.

OUR PRIORITIES AFTER OUR FAMILY

Where do our priorities lie outside the family? Who is our neighbour? Priorities, in a sense, take on a different aspect outside our family, where we are primarily concerned with our time and energies. The question should not be: *"Who is my neighbour?"* but, perhaps, as Jesus changed it to: *"To whom do I prove myself to be a neighbour?"* (Cf. Luke 10:36). Again, we must ensure that reaching out to others outside our family does not disorder our higher priorities for any significant period of time.

6. Gender Differences

'Male and female he created them.' (Genesis 1:27b)

We have picked out a number of areas in which the differences between the sexes may cause problems including, but not exclusively, brain differences. We must all be aware that basically, as men and women, our bodies are different and that those parts of the body that enable women to carry, give birth and nurture children are unique to them. Not so many may be aware of the fact that our 'wiring' is fundamentally different. As Moir & Jessel state in their book *Brainsex – The Real Difference Between Men and Women* (London: Mandarin Paperbacks, 1991): *"The way our brains are made affects how we think, learn, see, smell, feel, communicate, love, make love, fight, succeed, or fail."* Our brains have developed differently, as men and women, to enable us to successfully live and survive together. So where and why do difficulties occur?

TALKING AND LISTENING

In communication, these differences in our brain development can lead to frustration, misunderstanding and worse, if we don't accept them or recognise what is happening. Speech is not a specific brain skill for men and, accordingly, men's verbal abilities are inferior to women's, using about a third fewer words. In consequence, men are less descriptive but more direct, using the literal meaning of words. It results in sentences that are more structured and logical. Men, when presented with a problem, tend to 'talk' silently to themselves, thinking it over, and only resort to speech when they have arrived at a solution. Interruptions can cause them to become angry!

Women love talking and are great talkers. Speech is a specific area in the woman's brain; so, consequently, having these specific areas enables the woman's brain to be available for other tasks while speaking. This 'multitracking' ability enables women to speak and listen simultaneously, and to do this on several unrelated subjects. Men cannot speak and listen at the same time! Women use indirect speech, which means they hint in a roundabout way at what they want or mean, thus avoiding possible confrontation or aggression. This leaves men, who use direct speech, very confused and feeling they need to be mind-readers! Vocabulary is not a specific spot in the woman's brain, so the precise meanings of words are not important to her. Consequently exaggeration, emotive words, and using words she does not really mean, are generally part of her normal conversation. Women's brains are wired to use speech as the main form of expression, so they think aloud. When dealing with plans or problems, they will talk aloud about all the options, possibilities, what they need to do, to get, or where they need to go – and in no apparent order or logic.

If you are the husband you need to recognise that, when your wife is speaking her 'mind' at the end of the day, or whenever, she does not want interruptions with solutions to her problems. She will just want to be listened to, certainly empathically and sympathetically if appropriate, but not with *'Mr Fix-It' solutions!* With your logical and analytical brain you are always working out solutions to problems, so there is a constant danger that, if your wife talks about problems, you feel she expects you to solve them. This is not so - she just wants to talk it out! If she wants help, she will ask you for it, albeit indirectly! Under stress or pressure a woman's speech function will be activated and she will talk, often non-stop, to anyone who will listen,

about everything that is causing her the stress. She needs to be heard, above all, by you, but she doesn't want your solutions!

SPATIAL ABILITY

This is the ability is to be able to picture in the mind the shape of things, their dimensions, proportions, movement and geography. It also involves being able to imagine an object being rotated in space, navigating around an obstacle course, and seeing things from a three-dimensional perspective.

Spatial ability in men is a specific brain function located in the problem-solving area. In women, there is no specific location in the brain for this function; consequently, only about 10% of women have good or excellent ability in this area. Most men are good at activities that use spatial skills, and often pursue related careers such as motor mechanics, engineering, and airline flying and navigating. Women are noticeably absent in occupations requiring spatial ability.

Men, having good spatial abilities, are good map-readers and have a good sense of direction; moreover, they have the ability to store this information for future use. Men, for the same reason, are able to judge accurately whether an object will fit into a certain place or not, for example in the parallel parking of a car. Women tend to find these things very difficult if not impossible.

Our gender differences and their effects, as discussed above, are likely to be the cause of protests from feminists and politically correct activists, who might say that many of these matters are really the prejudices of society that reinforce stereotypical behaviours. Nevertheless, science has proved without doubt that our brains *are* different, and those differences give us advantages and disadvantages when compared with the opposite sex; however, there are always exceptions.

As spouses you need to be aware of these differences, and accept them if they apply in your own cases. Importantly, be sympathetic, understanding, and helpful where possible and appropriate; never be critical, impatient and rude, or ridicule your spouse. See and enjoy your differences!

MENSTRUAL CYCLE

While dealing with differences between men and women, the emotional highs and lows of the woman's menstrual cycle are important for all women and men to understand, especially husbands and wives. Pre-Menstrual Tension (PMT) is a major problem for modern women and one which her more ancient ancestors didn't have to deal with, as they tended to be pregnant or breast-feeding their children most of the time.

During the menstrual cycle the woman's mood and self-esteem are directly affected by the production of hormones, which fluctuate predictably during the twenty-eight-day cycle. At the time of menstruation, the hormone oestrogen is at its lowest level, as is the general 'mood' of the woman, who often feels depressed. However, the level increases over the next twenty-one days until it peaks near the time of ovulation at mid-cycle. This hormone creates feelings of well-being and happiness, and this is a time of greatest emotional optimism, self-confidence and self-esteem. This is also the time when the level of the hormone testosterone is highest, giving the woman a positive attitude to life with least anxiety. After ovulation the hormone progesterone is produced, bringing with it increasing tension, anxiety, and aggressiveness during the second half of the cycle. These two hormones decrease during the premenstrual period, reducing the mood to its lowest point again. This premenstrual phase is associated with feelings of helplessness, anxiety, hostility and yearning for love. The tension and the irritability ease at menstruation.

As the wife, it is vital for you to understand how the menstrual cycle impacts on your emotions. Whilst this will, of course, vary in intensity, it will always be present. Moreover, it will be superimposed over your 'current' emotional state resulting from your situation and circumstances at that particular time, which may alleviate or accentuate your feelings. It is important that you should interpret your feelings with caution and scepticism during your premenstrual period; and you should try to remember that the despair and sense of worthlessness you may experience are hormonally induced and have nothing to do with reality. Then you can better withstand the psychological nosedive more easily.

As the husband, it is equally important that you too understand the menstrual cycle and its effects, particularly recognising the emotional changes which will usually accompany it, in order that you can be sensitive, understanding and especially loving at this time. However, this needs to be subtle and not condescending, and remarks such as "it must be the wrong time of

the month", or similar, must be avoided at all costs.

THE MARITAL EMBRACE

In sexual intercourse a husband and wife give themselves to each other with the intention of procreation and personal unity, which makes conjugal love a mutual giving and receiving in a way that is physically, emotionally and spiritually satisfying for both spouses as sexually complementary beings. It aims at a deeply personal unity, a unity even beyond "the becoming one flesh", because it leads to the forming of *one heart and one soul.* Conjugal love, because it involves total self-surrender of spouses one to the other - who are procreative human beings open to fertility and life - demands a relationship that is total, exclusive, indissoluble and faithful till death. If any of these aspects are missing, the marriage can be in deep trouble. Cf. (CCC n.1643).

The physical joining in sexual intercourse should therefore be a sign and confirmation of your common life together. It consummates and embodies the words of love you expressed in the exchange of vows on your wedding day by which you both belong to each other until death parts

you. Clearly, *you renew these vows every time you have sexual intercourse.*

Sadly, this marital act frequently becomes a divisive factor in marriages, often leading to infidelity and break-up. So often this is due to a complete lack of knowledge or understanding of the *critical differences between men and women, in the area of sexuality, and the sensitivity it calls for.*

Firstly, then, let us look at the area of *sexual desire and stimulation,* which are very different in men and women. A failure to understand this uniqueness can produce a continual source of marital frustration and guilt. *Sexual desire* in females is usually correlated to the menstrual cycle, and this is obviously something that a husband needs to be aware of and understand about his wife. In a man, sexual desire occurs whenever he is appropriately stimulated. In turn, stimulation in men is primarily *visual.* Men tend to be turned on by feminine nudity or glimpses of semi-nudity. This stimulation is *sheer biological power resulting from physical, bodily attraction.*

Women are much more discriminating in their sexual interests, and tend to be more aroused by the romantic aura which surrounds the man, together with the man's character and personality. He must appeal to her both emotionally and physically. There must be affection, as well as physical closeness, before a woman may be ready to be stimulated by touch. The importance of these differences is that sex for a man is a more physical thing, while for a woman it is a deeply emotional experience. *This sexual distinction between men and women affects every act of love they make.*

As a husband you would wish and expect your wife to enjoy and respond to the sexual act as you do, but you may be aware that often she does not. However, bearing in mind the differences mentioned above, it is easy to see why this may be so. For your wife cannot enjoy it unless she feels you respect her, and are emotionally close to her at the time and, moreover, have been loving, tender and romantic before the encounter. So it is probable that she has not felt that you have been like that on those occasions. You probably may not have been aware of that, or may have thought that the sexual act would heal any slight upset between you. The solution to a happy sex life together is to try to apply romantic love to every aspect of your wife's existence, to build up her self-esteem, her joy in living, and her sexual responsiveness.

With this in mind, another important difference between men and women which needs to be understood in this area, particularly by husbands, is often known as the 'Gas Ring Principle'. *The sexual arousal of women may be likened to a ring on an electric hob.* Turned on, it takes a while before it really gets up to full temperature. Moreover, after it is turned off, it remains hot for five minutes or more! *Men, on the other hand, may be likened to a gas ring* - turn it on and it is ready. When turned off it dies and cools instantly. However, ideally, they need to achieve climax at the same time! It takes women much longer to get involved but, once they do, they feel like that for some time afterwards. Men, on the other hand, seem to function as if they are ready to go at a moment's notice, and equally ready to roll over and go to sleep when the act is finished. It is essential that spouses learn, with foreplay and patience, how to *reach climax together* if possible, otherwise the wife may be left completely aroused but unsatisfied. *The husband clearly has the responsibility to ensure this does not happen!* If a wife is continually left aroused, but not satisfied, she will inevitably begin to dislike sexual intercourse, to the detriment of the whole relationship.

The climax of the sexual act should reflect an ecstatic moment where the husband freely and unreservedly surrenders himself to his wife, and she freely and unreservedly receives him. For in sexual intercourse we are, in effect, saying with our bodies: *"I want to give myself to you, to affirm your goodness and our marriage commitment."* This is what Paul was implying in his Letter to the Thessalonians:

"For this is the will of God... that each one of you knows how to take a wife for himself in holiness and honour, not in the passion of lust like heathen who do not know God" (1 Thessalonians 4: 3-5)

What truly violates freedom in intercourse is where there is any manipulation or coercion between one spouse and the other. For example, when we use sex in our relationship as a tool, perhaps to gain power or control, or to offer it as a 'reward' for something else, or even withhold it as a 'punishment'. Freedom is also violated if sex is engaged in to meet a selfish, compulsive need for gratification; an extreme case of this would be *'marital rape'*. With our spouse, particularly in this area, *we should not be looking for what we can get out of the relationship*, but rather what we can put into it. Otherwise, this would mean that we see our spouse more as an *object* that can be used as a means to an end, rather than a *person* endowed with dignity by God to whom we wish to give our self.

Appendix

'Let the little children come to me, and do not hinder them, for the kingdom of heaven belongs to such as these.' Matthew 19:14 (NIV)

The process of 'Selective Intercourse', whereby couples choose which time of the woman's fertility cycle they wish to use, varies according to their intentions at the time. If a couple wish to conceive, they target intercourse during the fertile days; otherwise, they select the infertile days if they would prefer to avoid pregnancy. In most cases, a couple will use natural family planning only to limit the total number of children and to provide a space of time between births. They must have a just reason to do so, such as the limited resources of the family and the need to provide for existing children. It is immoral to attempt to use NFP so strictly as to eliminate the possibility of conception, that is, with a 'contraceptive mentality'. The couples' intentions must be open to life and to the will of God concerning the procreation of children. Cf. (CCC n.2366).

In *Familiaris Consortio* (n.32), Blessed Pope John Paul II states that "The choice of the natural rhythms involves accepting the cycle of the person, that is the woman, and thereby accepting dialogue, reciprocal respect, shared responsibility and self-control. To accept the cycle and to enter into dialogue means to recognise both the spiritual and corporal character of conjugal communion and to live personal love with its requirement of fidelity. In this context the couple comes to experience how conjugal communion is enriched with those values of tenderness and affection which constitute the inner soul of human sexuality, in its physical dimension also. In this way sexuality is respected and promoted in its truly and fully human dimension, and is never 'used' as an 'object' that, by breaking the personal unity of soul and body, strikes at God's creation itself at the level of the deepest interaction of nature and person."

Natural family planning, in using the natural increase and decrease in fertility built into a woman's menstrual cycle to increase or decrease the possibility of conception, requires accurate self-observation and recording. Several different modern methods are reliable, effective, respect the bodies of the spouses, and encourage tenderness between them. Cf. (CCC n.2370). The three methods described below have all been shown to be very accurate in interpreting the fertility cycle, providing the method is rigidly adhered to.

The **Billings Ovulation Method** uses observations about changes in a woman's body during her menstrual cycle to determine the time when she is most fertile. It is applicable from puberty to menopause, in times of breast-feeding, and post-hormonal medication. It can be used to achieve or avoid pregnancy. Cycles do not have to be regular. It is based on symptoms of fertility and infertility. Mucus that is produced at the cervix is felt by a woman at the vulva as she goes about her daily activities. There is no need for her to touch the mucus, but the sensation and appearance help her to identify the fertile and infertile times in her cycle, and the time of ovulation. This is achieved by keeping a record of the sensation and appearance of the mucus at the vulva at the end of each day, on a special chart.

The **Creighton Model System** is a modified version of the Billings Ovulation Method, and is effective for every kind of cycle: long, short, irregular, post-hormonal medication, peri-menopause, or during breast-feeding. The System relies upon the standardized observation and charting of external observations of the discharge of the cervical mucus, the presence of bleeding and the days when no discharge is present (dry days), all of which are used to obtain pertinent information on the phases of fertility and infertility to either achieve or avoid pregnancy. Users of CrMS know their fertility status on any particular day and are given the freedom to utilize that information as they so choose. The biomarkers used can also help to identify abnormalities in a woman's health. If there are any specific problems (usually related to fertility issues), they can be addressed using NaPro Technology, which is the new, ethical health science that works cooperatively with a woman's cycle and nature.

The **Symptothermal Method** requires the woman to learn about her body's natural fertility signs and take her temperature every morning. Daily temperature readings are performed using a **basal thermometer,** a special thermometer that will determine the body's temperature within a few hundredths of a degree. This level of precision is necessary to detect the slight temperature increase that marks the end of the fertile period. The woman keeps a chart where she records her daily temperature and also other body signs that indicate when ovulation will occur. Other body signs include cervical mucus consistency, cervical position, mid-cycle cramping, and mood. To use this method, couples need to receive training from a certified natural family planning instructor.

If you wish for more information on these three methods, the following websites provide the details, diagrams, and charts necessary to understand and carry out the procedures and observations necessary for that particular method.

BILLINGS OVULATION METHOD (BOM)
http://www.billingsnaomi.org

This is a UK site providing information packs, charts and learning materials. Instruction can also be given. There is a link included to the international Billings website: Billings LIFE.

CREIGHTON MODEL (CrMS)
http://www.lifefertilitycare.co.uk

This is the UK site of Life Fertility Care Clinic providing explanation of the method, articles and videos and, importantly, relates the method to the spirit of Blessed John Paul II's "inner soul of human sexuality". The system requires initial practitioner support for proper use, and enquiry forms are included.

SYMPTOTHERMAL METHOD (STM)
http://www.fertilityet.org.uk

This site provides excellent on-line tutorials with illustrations and charts to enable step-by-step charting of your fertility cycle. The *Couple to Couple League* organisation runs 3-session STM courses at various venues in the UK, as well as providing a Home Study course. Resources and materials are obtainable online at: http://www.cclgb.org.uk